Shine Like a Mother

6 Steps for Thriving After C-Section

Natalie Miller, MOT, OTR/L, PCES

SHINE LIKE A MOTHER

Dedicated to my family and friends who are like family. Thank you for supporting me in so many ways during this journey.

ACKNOWLEDGMENTS

I want to first acknowledge my parents for teaching me how to be independent, resilient, and creative. You gave me the wings I needed to fly.

Thank you to my husband, Daniel, and kids, Dylan and Teagan, for standing by me and believing in me and all of my ideas. You inspire me to be better and remind me that I can figure things out.

I also want to thank my OT professors, colleagues, and supervisors who have modeled incredible professional and interpersonal skills and motivated me to grow beyond where I saw myself when I was first starting out.

Finally, thank you to all of my friends who patiently listened to my ideas, gave suggestions, and encouraged me throughout the process of writing a book. It takes a village, and I am so grateful.

NATALIE MILLER

A NOTE TO THE READER

Natalie Miller, the author of this C-section wellness guide, is the founder and owner of mighty mOThers, LLC, a small practice that serves pregnant and postpartum moms. She has a license and 15 years of experience as an occupational therapist.

OTs are board-certified health professionals trained by accredited higher learning institutions in anatomy and physiology, human development, mental health, neuroanatomy, and more. They serve a variety of populations and are highly skilled at breaking down barriers within tasks, routines, and environments to make them not only manageable, but enjoyable. Occupations refer to the preferred everyday activities that make a person an individual (and don't always have to be paid jobs!)

OTs have the option to do additional advanced trainings and become specialists in certain areas of healthcare, including things like wound care, lymphedema management, and brain injury treatment. Natalie has taken courses in maternal health, trauma-informed care, scar management, myofascial release, and Kinesiotape application, and is a certified Pregnancy and Postpartum Corrective Exercise Specialist. Expertise and experience in maternal health and rehabbing the body and mind were used to create a wellness guide just for you.

While the information contained within this guide relates to health issues, the contents are not a substitute for medical or health advice from a professional who is aware of the facts and circumstances of your individual situation. mighty mOThers, LLC, expressly recommends that you seek advice from a professional, and someone who knows about YOU.

The content within this wellness guide and the resources available for download through our website are not intended as, and shall not be understood or construed as, medical advice. All content has the intent to be informational and supportive.

We have done our best to ensure that the information provided within this guide is accurate and valuable.

Neither mighty mOThers, LLC, nor any of its employees or owners shall be held liable or responsible for any errors or omissions within this guide or for any damage you may suffer as a result of failing to seek competent medical or health advice from a professional who is familiar with your situation. Thank you.

NATALIE MILLER

CONTENTS

1   Know the Nitty-Gritty of Your Surgery   3

2   Take Care of Your Healing Scar   19

3   Learn Ergonomics & Functional Momming   27

4   Get Tools for Healing After C-section   43

5   When All Else Fails, Breathe   53

6   Set Goals and Expectations for YOU   67

7   A Few Final Thoughts   75

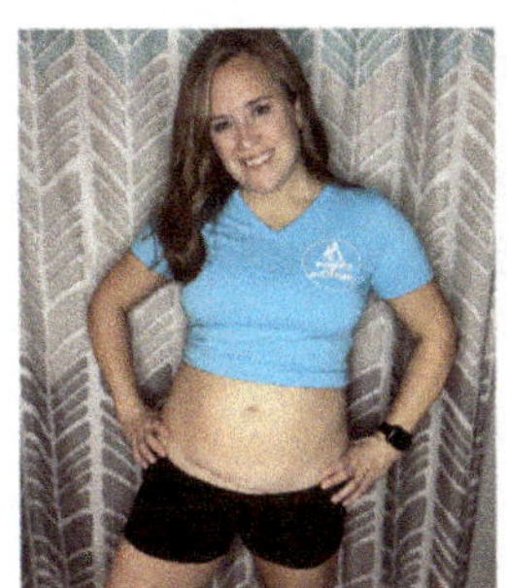

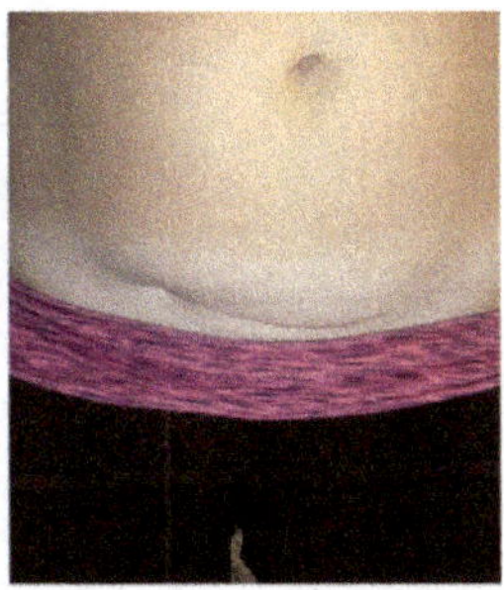

NATALIE MILLER

1
KNOW THE NITTY-GRITTY OF YOUR SURGERY

You are the only person who has EVER lived in your own body. You are the only one who has ever, and will ever, feel the physical and mental sensations that you feel, in the way you feel them. You are the only YOU who has been through the specific events and experiences that led you to where you are now in your life. Let that thought fully absorb! No one else can ever truly know your lived experience with the intimacy that you know it. Therefore, it truly wouldn't be a fair analogy if you were to compare yourself with a single other person or mama (although most of us do this on the regular anyway!) The type of birth you had is no exception to this.

My number one recommendation for you is to try your best to avoid the comparison game with your birth story and healing process because there truly is only one exact example: your own!

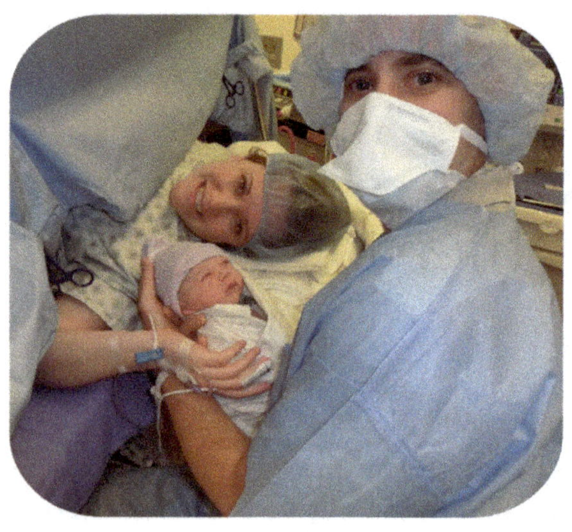

In this photo, you see a glimpse into my first birth story – but remember, it's only an instant in time. I look happy, but I'm pretty sure that's mostly from the laughing gas I begged for! I had not anticipated or planned for a C-section at all and was terrified for what was to come with my own recovery. Of course, I was excited to meet my son, too. So many mixed emotions!

Now let's touch on the surgery itself before we go on to considerations for physical, mental, and functional recovery.

During the pregnancy phase, a lot of moving and stretching takes place (like a LOT!) Hormones play a part in the changes in how your body is functioning - they relax the ligaments in your pelvis, soften and widen the cervix, and change your skin's elasticity. It takes time for these things to work their way back toward their pre-baby ways. In the meantime, you may experience aches and pains, stretchy and loose-feeling body parts, and the effects of being on an emotional roller coaster.

Then, when baby is delivered via Cesarean, lots of layers of tissue have to be cut, manipulated, stretched, moved, and put back together to help baby come into the world.

There are 7 layers of tissue that have to be cut into and/or moved in order to access your baby safely. SEVEN!! Check out the photo below, because sometimes a visual can really help with processing things. This visual may also help provide you validation and help show others why the healing phase for your own body is so tough and so important. Your body and your healing are incredible! You deserve to have information and feel empowered about how to help yourself heal.

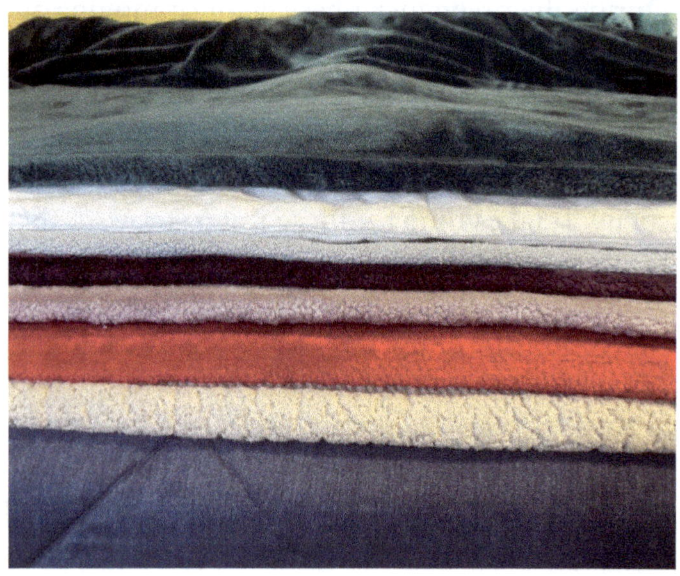

Here is the order of tasks the doctor will do[1]:

1. Cut through the skin (most of the time horizontally, in a little smiling line in the bikini area; sometimes in a vertical line but this is rare)

2. Cut through adipose (otherwise known as fatty tissue)

3. Cut through fascia (this stuff surrounds and supports all of your organs and other internal body parts)

4. Separate the abdominal muscles (they are not actually cut apart in the majority of cases - just gently separated right down their midline)

5. Cut through the peritoneum (a thin layer right before you get to the uterus)

6. Cut into the uterus

7. Open the amniotic sac (and gently take out baby!)

1. Source: Cesarean Section, https://www.ncbi.nlm.nih.gov/books/NBK546707/

Step 1: Cut horizontally through skin

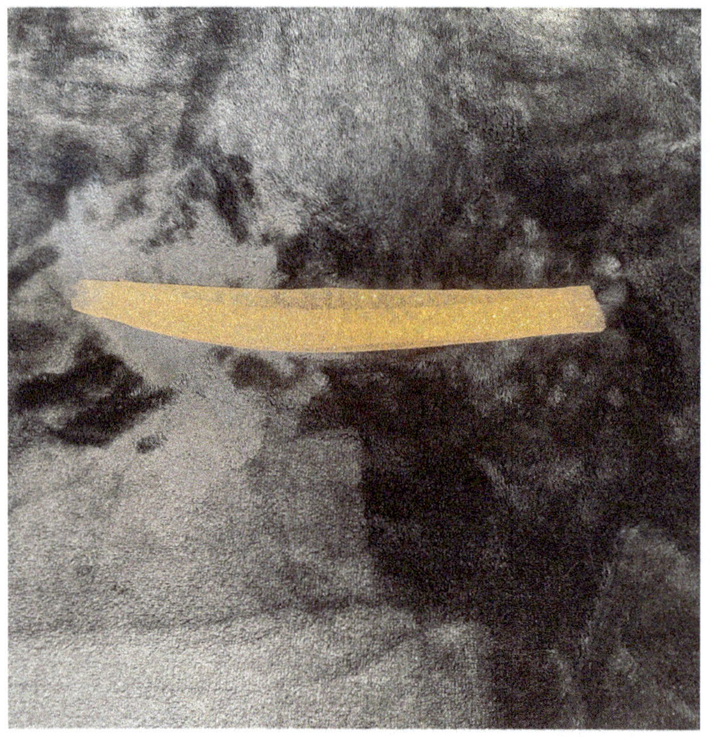

{On very rare occasions,
cut is vertical}

Step 2: Cut through adipose (fatty) tissue

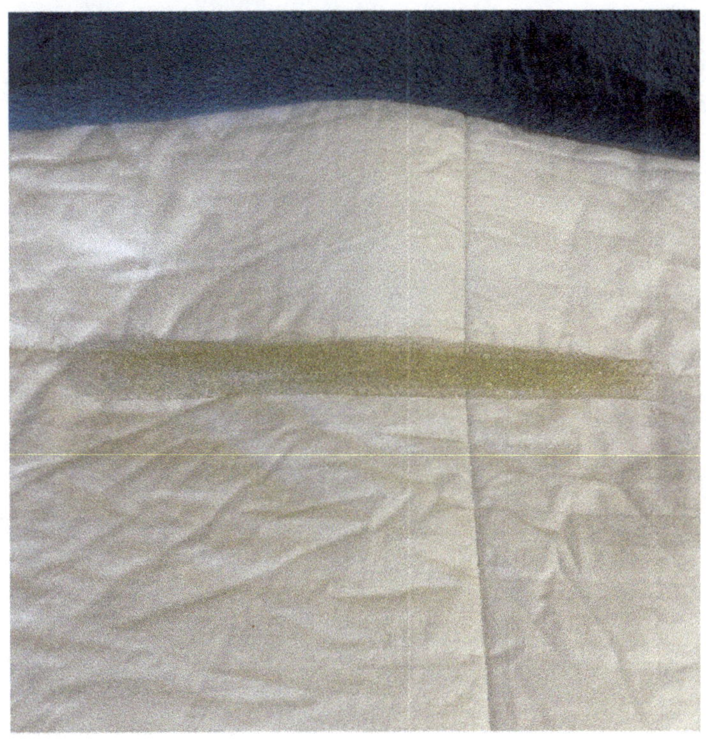

Step 3: Cut through fascia

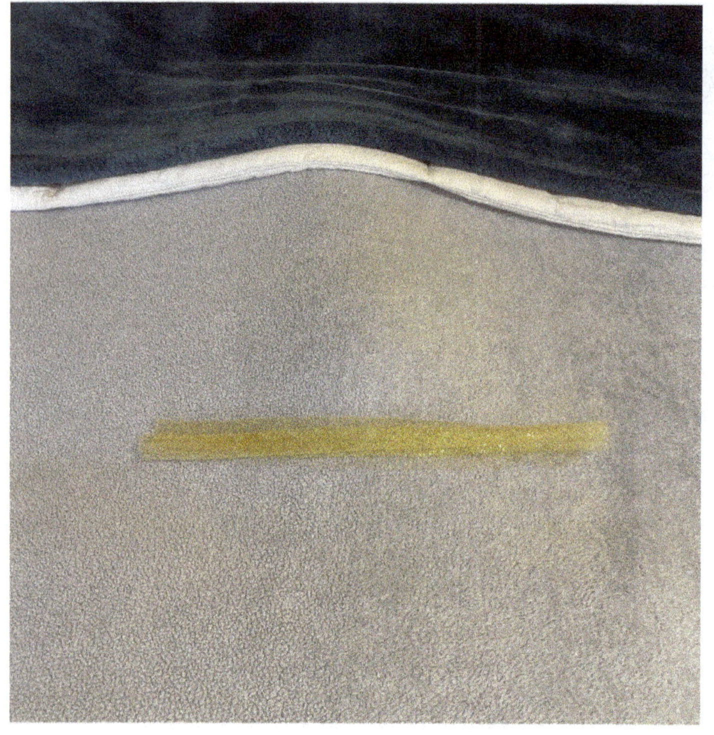

{This has nerves and feeling!}

Step 4: Separate abdominal muscles

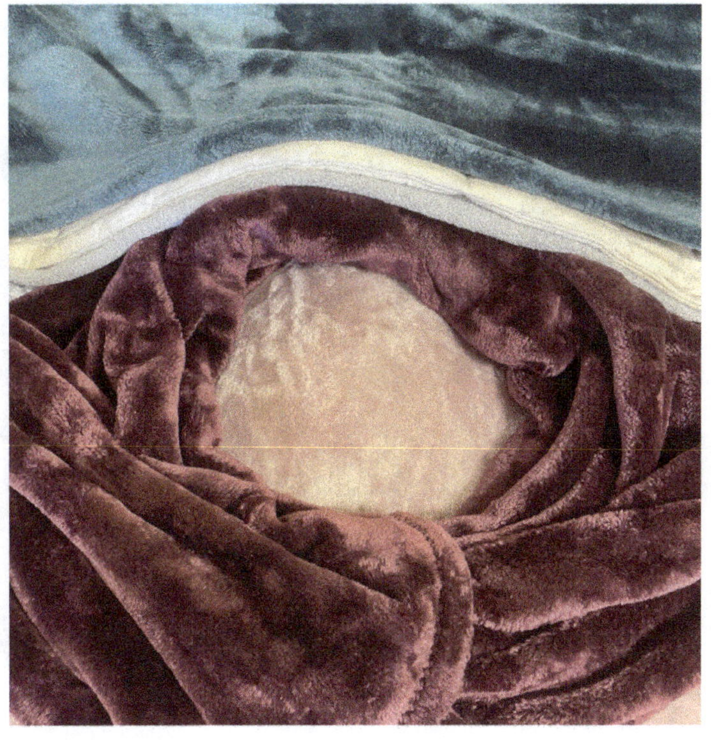

{Typically muscles aren't actually cut}

Step 5: Cut vertically through peritoneum

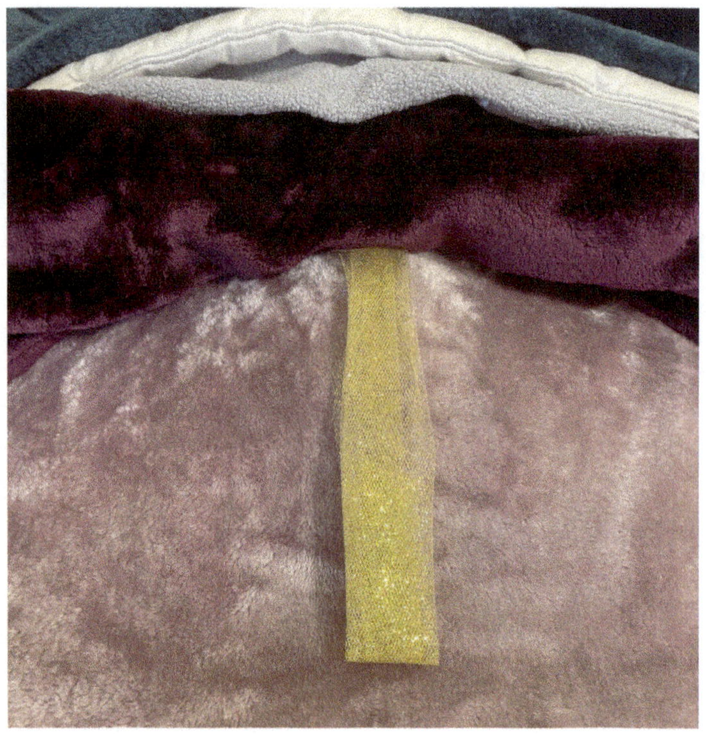

Step 6: Cut through uterus

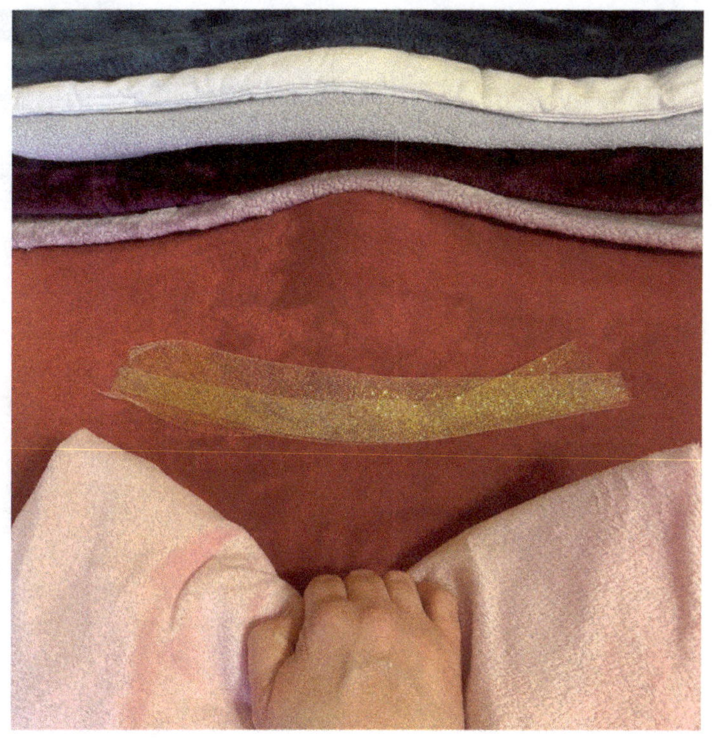

{Bladder is gently pushed down/out of the way}

Step 7: Cut into amniotic sac

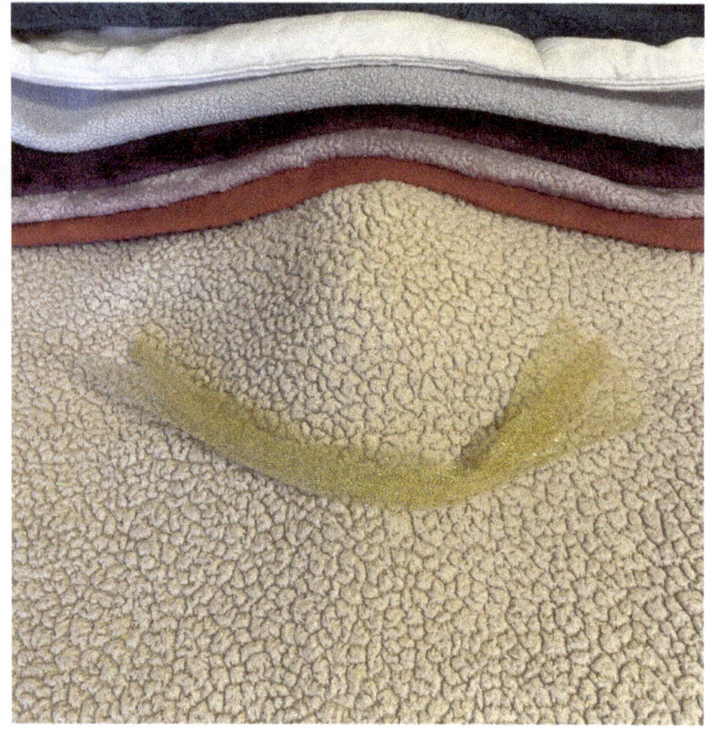

Out comes baby!

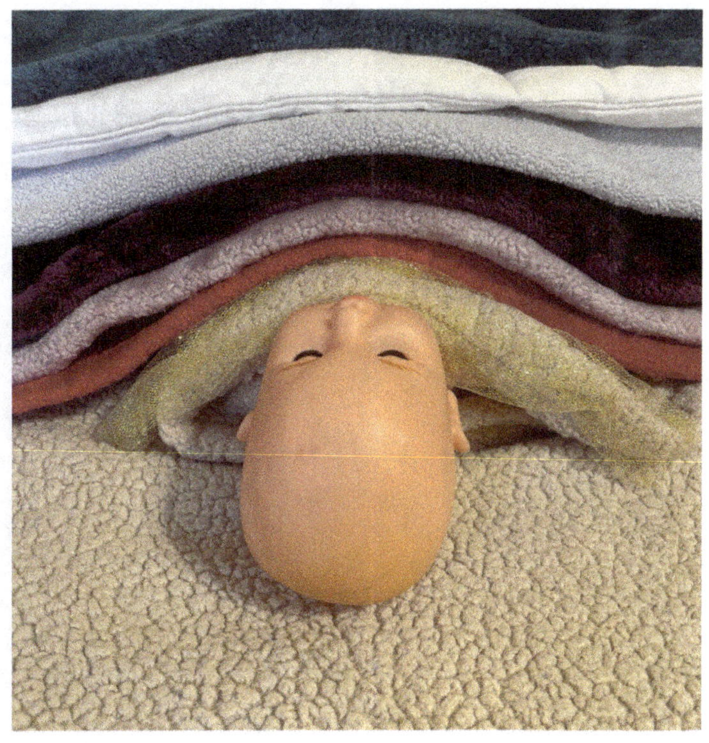

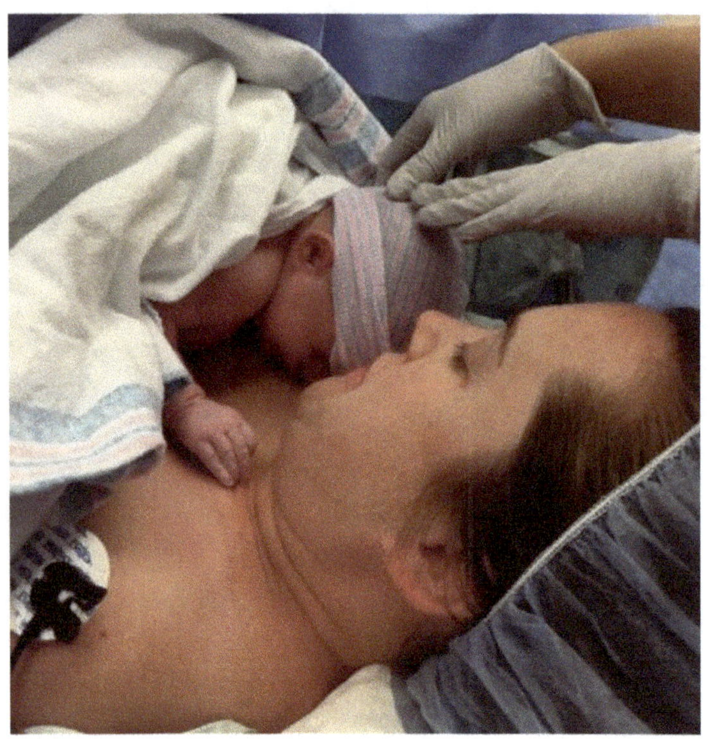

As you can imagine, this is why, even though muscle is not {typically} formally cut into, it takes quite a while for things to start to heal. AND this is why healing should be done in a careful, safe way, to help you be as strong and healthy as you can be months, and years, down the road.

In addition to the steps listed above, you also have to deal with a spinal or epidural for anesthesia, (or possibly even general anesthesia, depending on the severity of your situation) medications via IV, possibly oxygen through a mask or nasal cannula, and a Foley catheter inserted to help your bladder. That's a lot of things happening to one body, that don't even take into consideration the effects of pain, sleep deprivation, medications, worry, and hormones.

Keep in mind, too, that women have C-sections for many different reasons. In addition to going through a host of physical aspects of surgery, mamas are often going through a spectrum of emotional and mental healing. This also takes time, as any major transition does.

Off the top of my head, there is no other surgery this major that doesn't result in some type of rehabilitation or therapy program afterward to help folks get stronger and back on their feet. Most of the time, major surgeries involve multiple follow-ups with doctors, appointments with therapists, and intensive rehab protocols and exercises.

You are now trying to figure all of this out, plus all of your newborn's needs, while on very little sleep and with fluctuating hormones - mostly on your own, without the support listed above. But you deserve guidance and support. You deserve validation. Try to be gentle and kind to yourself during the weeks, months, and even years following your C-section delivery. You had a REAL birth. Don't ever let anyone make you feel otherwise.

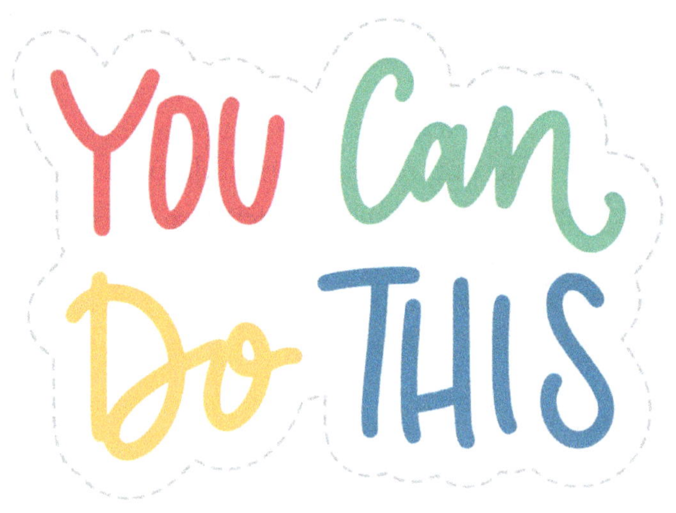

2
TAKE CARE OF YOUR HEALING SCAR

The scar that you are left with after your C-section is a beautiful reminder of the special journey you and your little one are on, but it may be painful, sensitive, and/or numb for weeks or months. It does serve a purpose - it is your body's way of patching up the hole that was created to get your baby out - but it can cause a range of discomfort and functional problems.

It's super important to try to keep the scar mobile so that it doesn't try to stick down internally to your organs or pull your posture downward as it tries to stick around the outer skin. The good news is that there are things that can be done that aren't too hard!

Step 1:
Wait about 2 weeks before worrying about touching it. In this timeframe, get used to looking at it, note changes, and get more comfortable seeing it. If you notice things that look worse (more swelling, redness, discharge, pain, funny smells, or you have a fever), putting in a call to your provider is a good idea. It is ok to take some time to adjust to your scar. It is a brand-new part of your body, and often it becomes a part of your life unexpectedly. Part of that adjustment is actually seeing it on yourself, little by little.

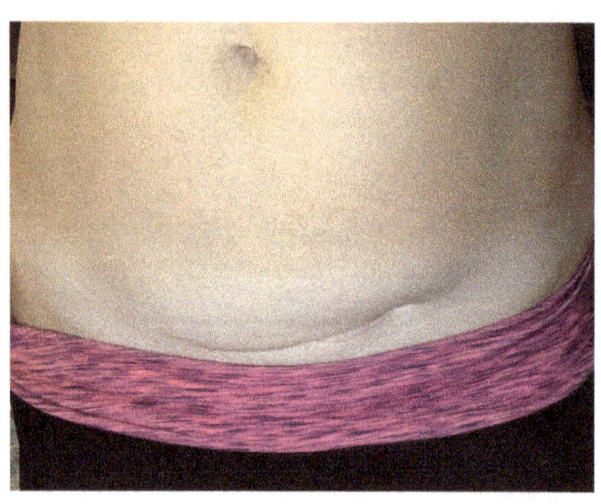

Step 2:

(Approximately weeks 2-6+) Start working on desensitization. This means you'll be getting your skin around the scar used to different sensory inputs, which will help it to adjust to feeling more "normal" things, like water spraying near it, clothes pulling up or down around it, or baby accidentally kicking or swiping near it.

Grab something soft (ideas: cotton balls, a small corner of fleece fabric), and make gentle, slow circles all around the scar - stay about 1-2 inches away from the actual scar, especially until it is fully healed. Do this 2-3 times a day for a few minutes at a time.

Start to progress what textures you feel ok with - maybe something slightly rougher or harder (ideas: paper towel, tissue paper, rougher washcloth). Continue 2-3 times a day but see if you can gradually increase how many minutes (maybe before you could do 2, now see if you can do 3-4).

Progress yourself even more with textures as you become more comfortable with the previous ones (ideas: denim, Velcro). Continue to progress either the amount of time you are able to do your circles, or how frequently you do these exercises.

Remember: you are in control of your own movements. If it is super uncomfortable at first, do it very briefly, or go farther away from the scar and inch your way closer. Remember not to go directly over your healing, new scar, especially with materials that could get stuck (like cotton balls)

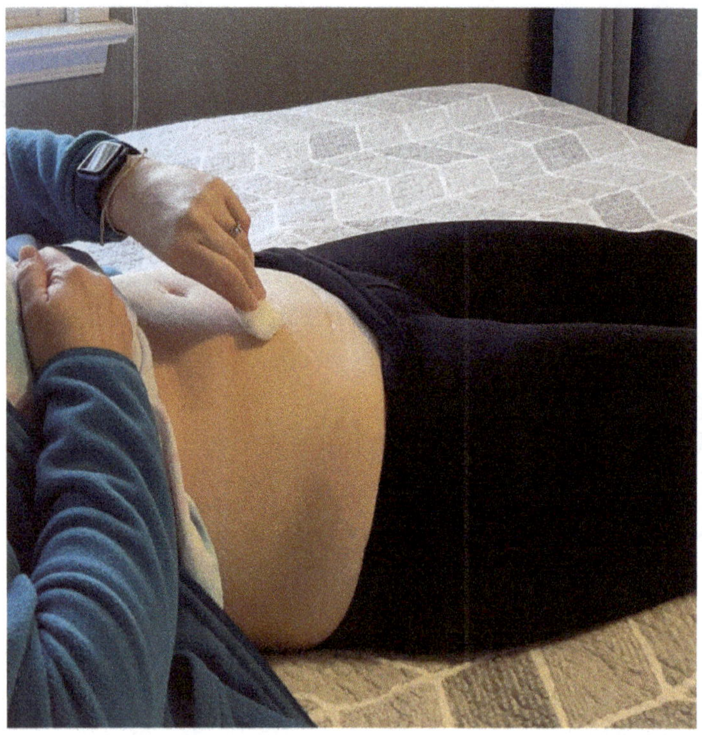

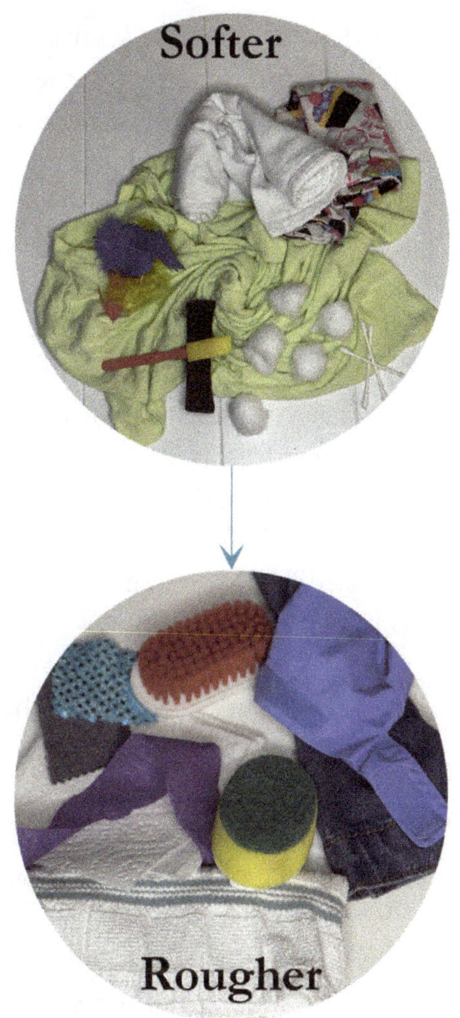
Softer
Rougher

Step 3:
Once your doctor has seen your scar around the 6-week mark and has given you the all-clear that things are healed (remember, this can be slightly longer for some women, and that's ok - stick to the desensitization until you are given the "A-Okay!"), you can move on to scar massage and mobilization.

This follows a very similar pattern as desensitization: start with a few minutes 2-3 times a day and progress yourself as you can a few more minutes, or more frequently. Start farther away from the scar (1-2 inches), and gradually get closer to it. Remember that scar tissue forms in all directions, so you'll want to vary the approach you take to help it move around more!

Take 2 fingers together and put them on your skin. With gentle but firm pressure, move your fingers around in little circles. Then move those fingers slightly to one side and do the circles again. Go all around the scar area; top, bottom, and sides. Change it up from little circles to zigzags or sideways movements. Again, you are in control here, so if it is too intense, lighten your touch a little bit! You can use lotion to help your fingers glide better if you'd like.

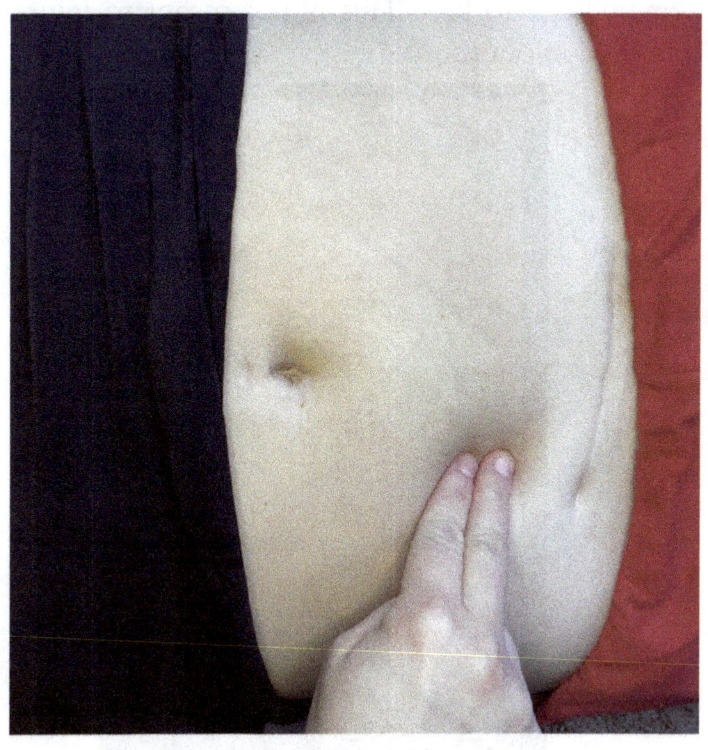

Follow up any desensitization or massage sessions with a few very gentle stretches. Sit on the ground and sway side to side with your arms in the air, like a tree branch swaying in the wind. Reach up to the sky, then slowly reach forward toward your feet. Turn your body slowly from side to side (like you are looking over your shoulder). Just like before, do all of this to tolerance - if you feel pain or pulling, do less! This is not meant to injure or stress you out more.

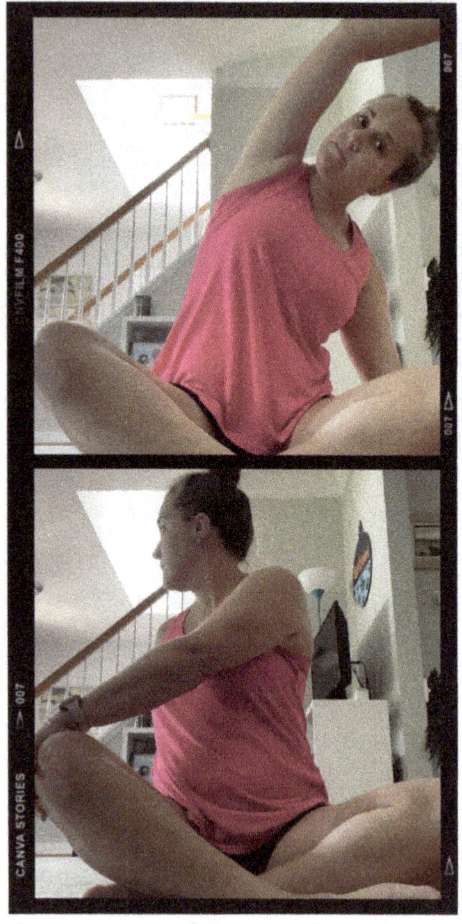

Keep that scar mobile so that down the road you'll have fewer complications and better overall mobility!

3
LEARN ERGONOMICS & FUNCTIONAL MOMMING

As humans, we are occupational beings - that means we thrive when we have a purpose, feel productive, and participate in our homes and communities. Even though you've had major surgery and welcomed a small, cute, (but needy) human into the world, your humanness and need/desire for function don't stop! It is possible to find ways to save your energy, avoid pain, and still participate meaningfully in your own life (as well as the life of your baby) despite and during your physical and emotional recovery.

To start with the physical aspect, don't be afraid to prioritize strategies that prevent or help take away pain, as well as save your energy. After all, it's pretty hard to function OR care for someone else (let alone a tiny infant) when you are in pain or overdoing things.

First up: the Log Roll. Get to know it and love it! When getting in and out of bed, move your shoulders, hips, and knees as one unit, and roll like a log. You may need to reach to the side of the bed with your hands, push up on your hands/elbows, and "hook" onto the bed with the backs of your legs. Just remember, use your hands, arms, and legs together, so that your healing abs don't get stuck with all of the workload. By doing this technique, you're protecting your surgical area, but still giving your abs a little chance to fire away and get stronger.

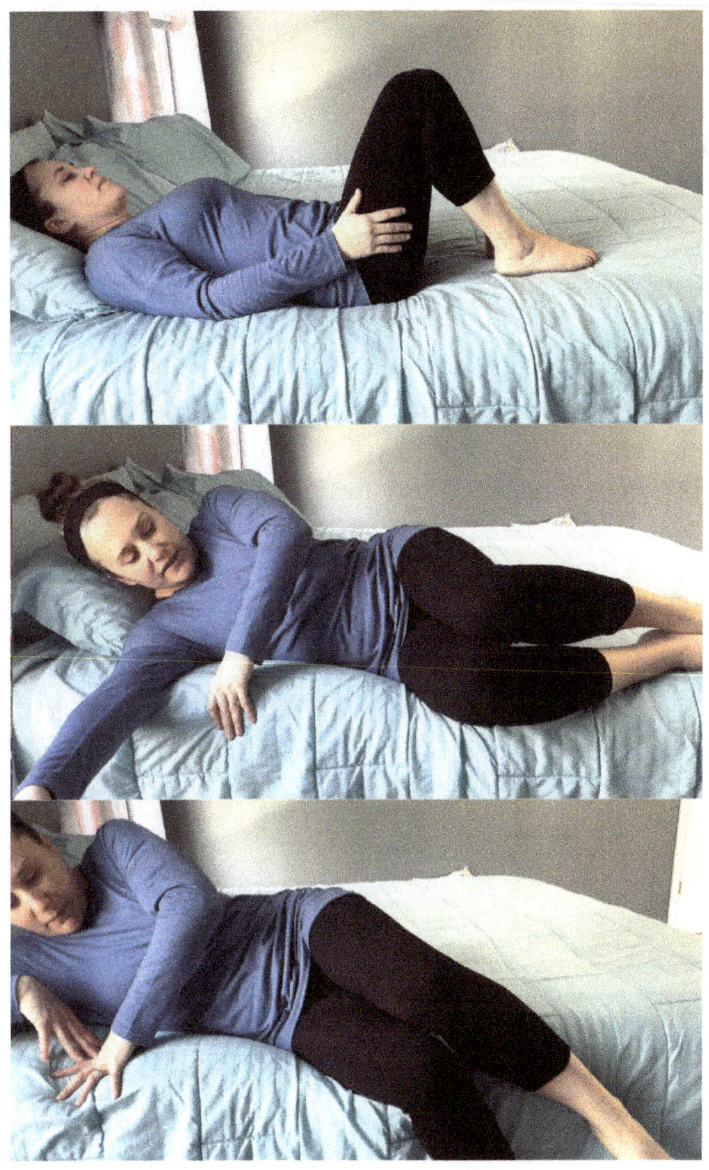

Next, Your position and setup matter. Often when we are doing things to help baby (such as feeding, changing diapers, bathing, even cuddling), we get into funky positions that don't necessarily serve our own bodies. Sometimes we do this because we're in a rush to get baby comforted, or feel a sense of urgency, or just because of habit. Our shoulders get hunched and/or tense, our bums are tucked under us, and our heads/necks are pointed downward. This can get pretty uncomfortable pretty quickly, and adds to strain in the neck, back, arms - and, heck, everywhere - over time.

Try to avoid this, at least sometimes!

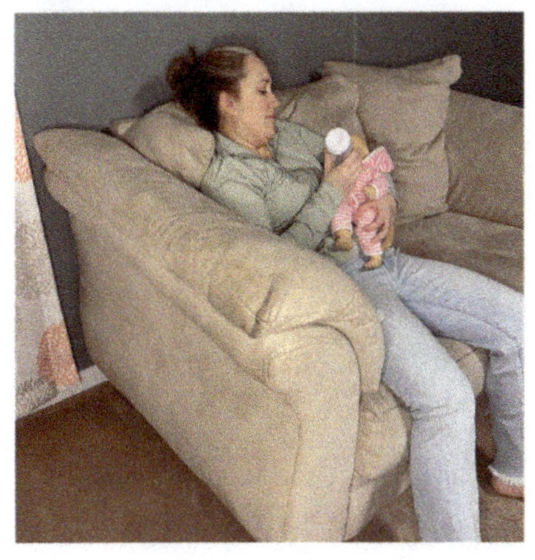

Try this instead!

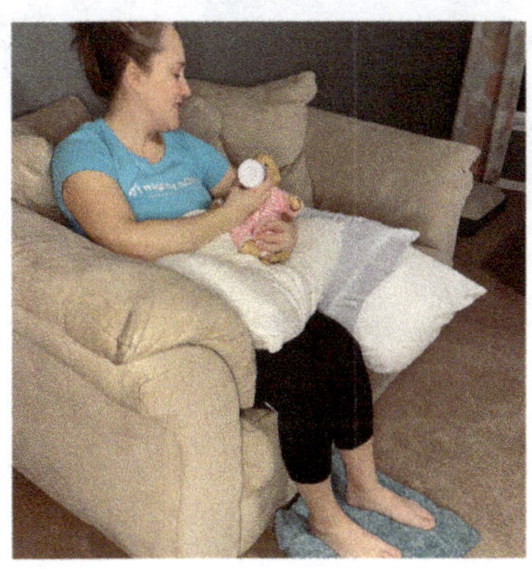

This is ok, but tough on the back and core

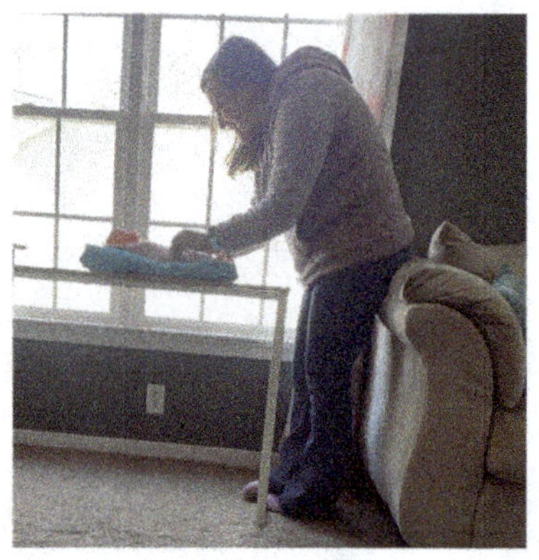

Try these instead!

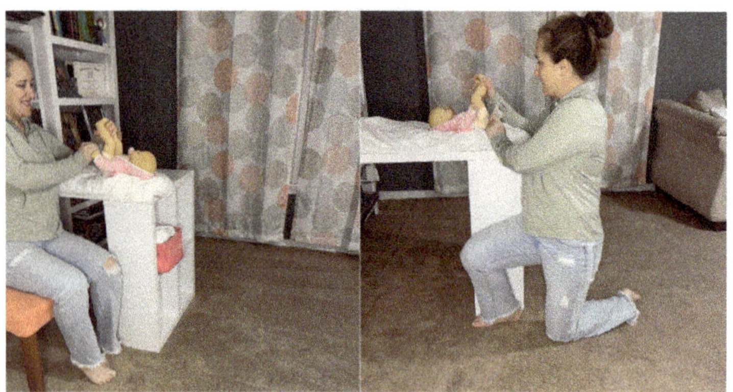

Try to take just a few moments ahead of your momming task to get yourself set up for success first. That might mean supporting your arms or lower back with a few pillows or a towel roll. Maybe it means putting a stool under your feet so they don't dangle and stress your lower back. Think about the position of your hands and wrists when you go to reach for baby, or a baby-related item (a bottle, stroller handle, baby carrier, etc.) and see if you can keep them in a neutral position (wrists not folded too far forward or backward) or if you can change up the position you use for these tasks to avoid overuse injury (can you sit down or kneel?).

While recovering from your surgery, your position matters even more. The more hunched over you are, the less gentle stretch and movement your scar area gets. You don't need to crank on it, but gently sitting up tall, or shifting in your seat, can go a long way toward allowing your scar to be more mobile.

Another idea to consider is setting up stations, or kits, of items you need for various mom tasks. This is also something awesome to ask for help with when visitors want to do something for you! Bottle/breast/pump feeding stations, toilet hygiene stations, diapering stations, you name it! Grab a small canvas or plastic tote and gather items you find yourself using frequently. That way, you can more gently reach toward what you need nearby, rather than needing to bend, lift, and twist. These more "torque-y" movements can put a lot of strain on your scar, and cause pain, so get yourself set up to avoid them.

While you are healing from a C-section, you are often told to avoid lifting anything that weighs more than the baby - well, what about the carrier? Groceries? Your toddler?! Here are some considerations to help you get things accomplished in spite of this weight-lifting restriction.

Consider:
- Sitting down for some activities (can you pull up a chair near your sink while you wash dishes or do laundry?)
- Sliding heavier objects on counters instead of lifting with your arms (place a hot pot on a trivet and slide it along the counter to your sink to dump the water)
- Using the stroller in your house to push baby around (or heavy items when baby is NOT in the stroller!)

- Prioritizing - make a list of what MUST be done and get that stuff done first - the rest can wait

- Following your body - if it hurts, slow down or do it differently (or not at all, right then - remember, you can always try again in a few days or a week)

- Teaching your toddler to do things with slightly more independence: crawling up into the car seat with your hand behind for guidance/support, stepping onto a stool to climb into bed with your hand behind for guidance/support, etc)

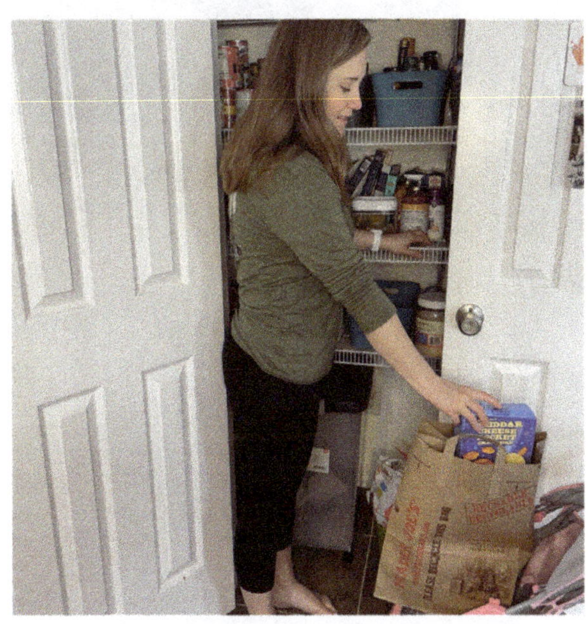

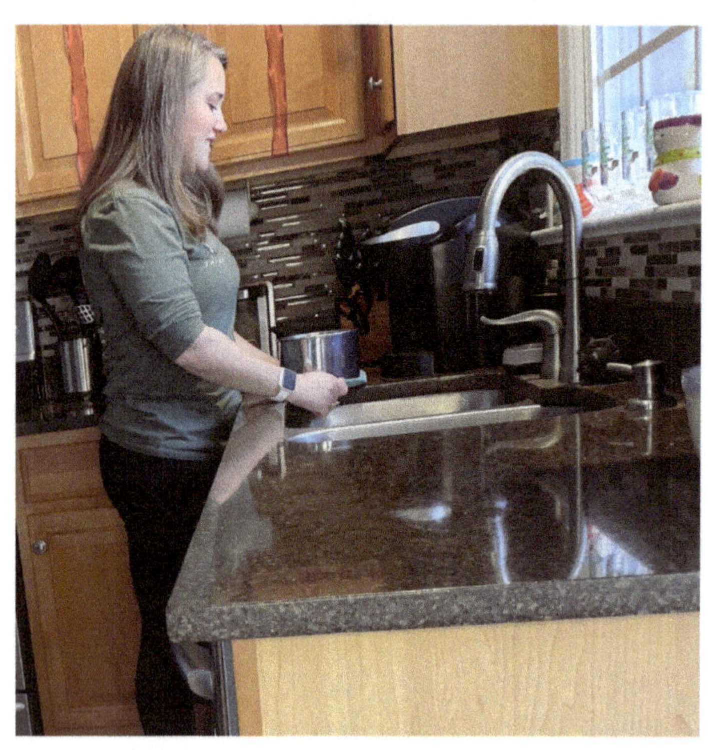

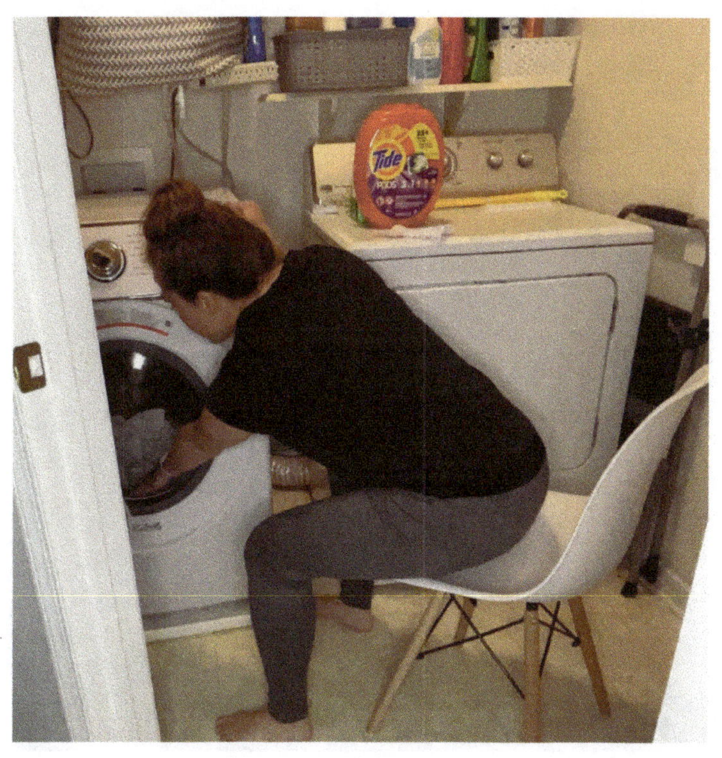

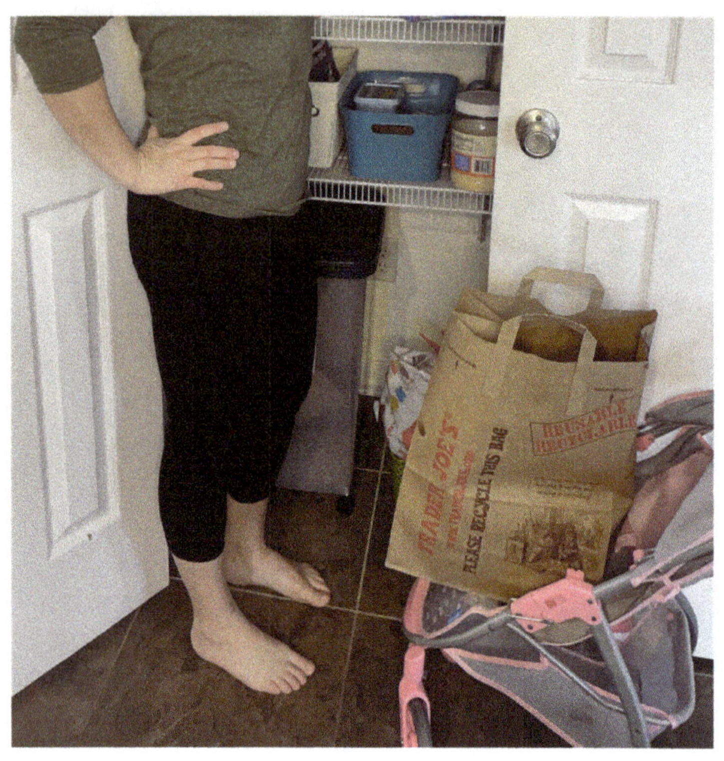

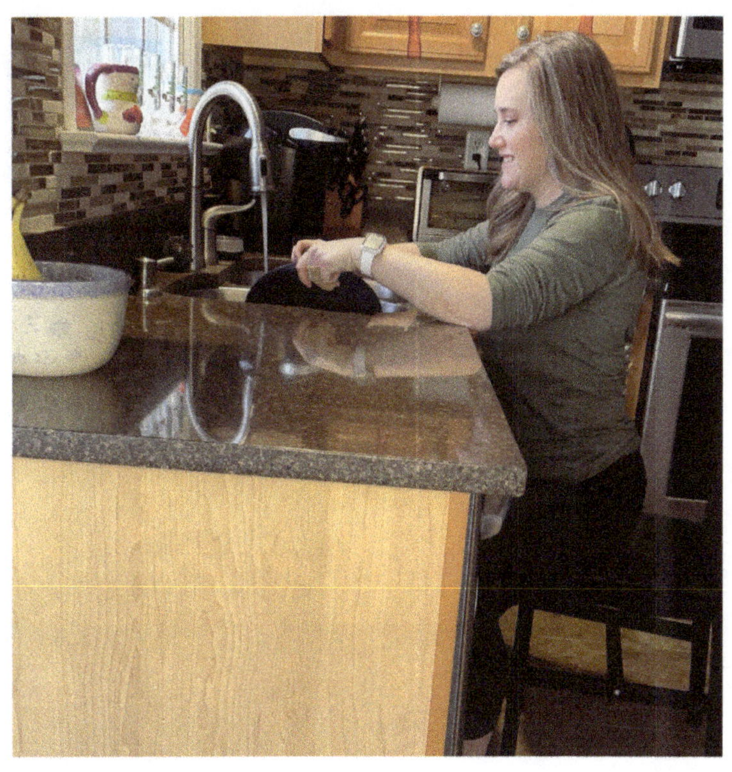

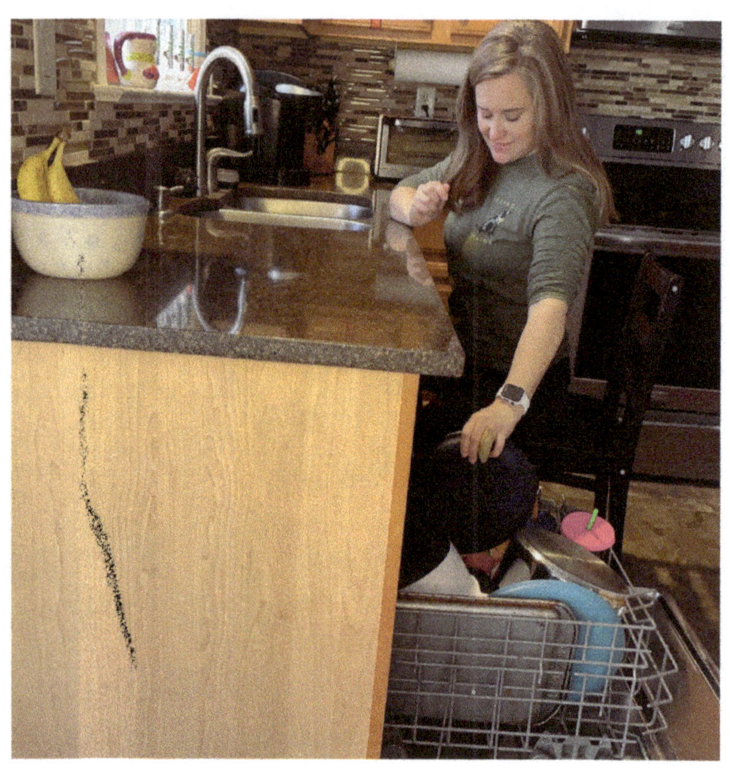

Thinking about and setting your intention each day will go far in helping you prevent and manage pain, protect your "you-ness," and truly set the tone for you being a functional, happy person and mama. You can do the things you want - you just may have to approach them a little bit differently.

42

4

GET TOOLS FOR HEALING AFTER A C-SECTION

There are lots of super helpful, super available items out there that can help you do things with less pain, help your surgical area heal, prevent issues with your scar and pelvic floor, and save you energy during the day.

Check out some common retailers for these items - Amazon, Walmart, and Target will probably have what you need! If not, you can always improvise with things you already have in your house (explanations on how are shown below.)

Handheld Shower Head:

There are a bunch of options that can be found on Amazon and Walmart.com - whether you want the cheap and easy install, or a more bougie look, do what makes you and your budget happy! Using this tool, you can more easily aim the stream of water so it doesn't directly flow on your incision area, since it's usually better for healing for water to drip slowly and less directly over it. This feels better, too, since direct streams of water can feel intense to those confused nerve endings. It can also help you to reach and more thoroughly wash areas such as your privates and feet without having to bend and twist (thus putting less strain on your healing scar!) Consider using a cup to pour water if you do not have access to a handheld shower head.

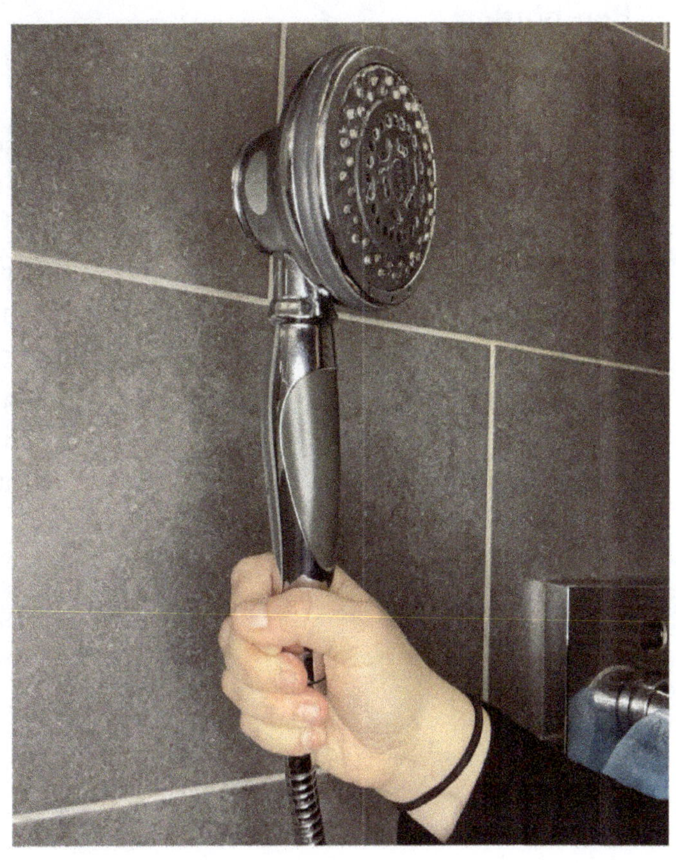

Peri bottle:

You can often get one of these during your hospital stay. Fill it with lukewarm water and use it to clean your private areas after going to the bathroom. Sometimes it's hard to reach when wiping due to your incision being sore, and this is more gentle and aimed directly where you need to be cleaned. Nurses often also suggest gently squeezing the water on yourself as you urinate, to take the sting away. Other options for this tool in a pinch: dollar bin squeeze bottles, or emptied (and thoroughly cleaned!!) contact solution bottles.

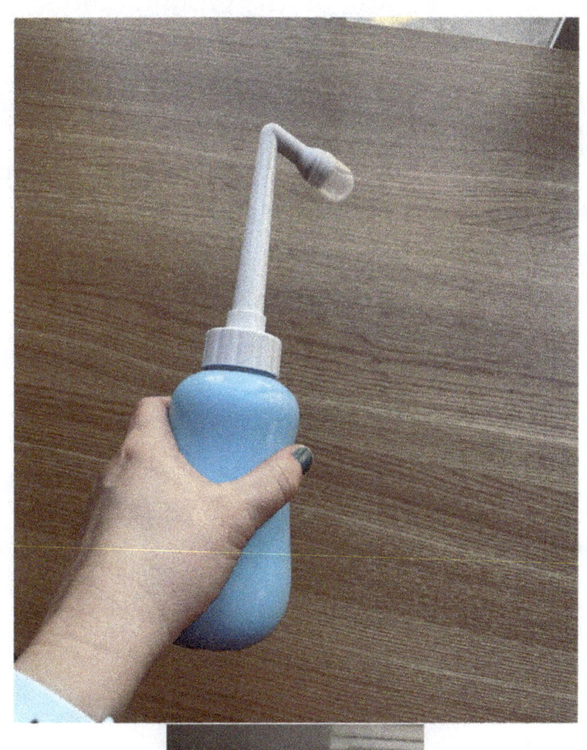

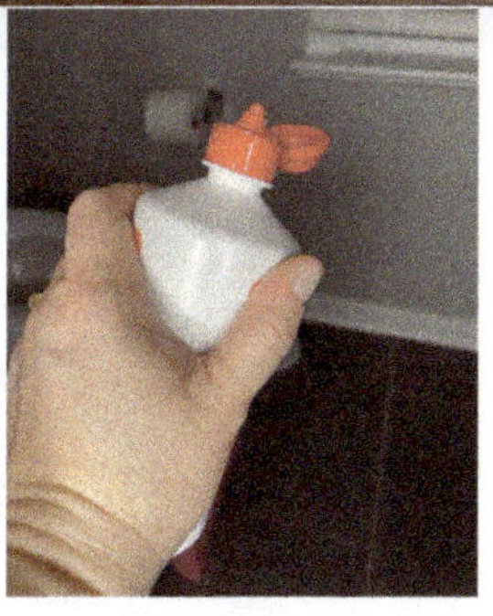

Yoga blocks:

You can place these on the ground (and stack as many as needed - I use 2, usually) to help position your bum in better alignment for less back strain and pain. This also helps you relax your abdomen and pelvic floor. Two or three towel rolls or smaller pillows stacked on each other will also do the trick.

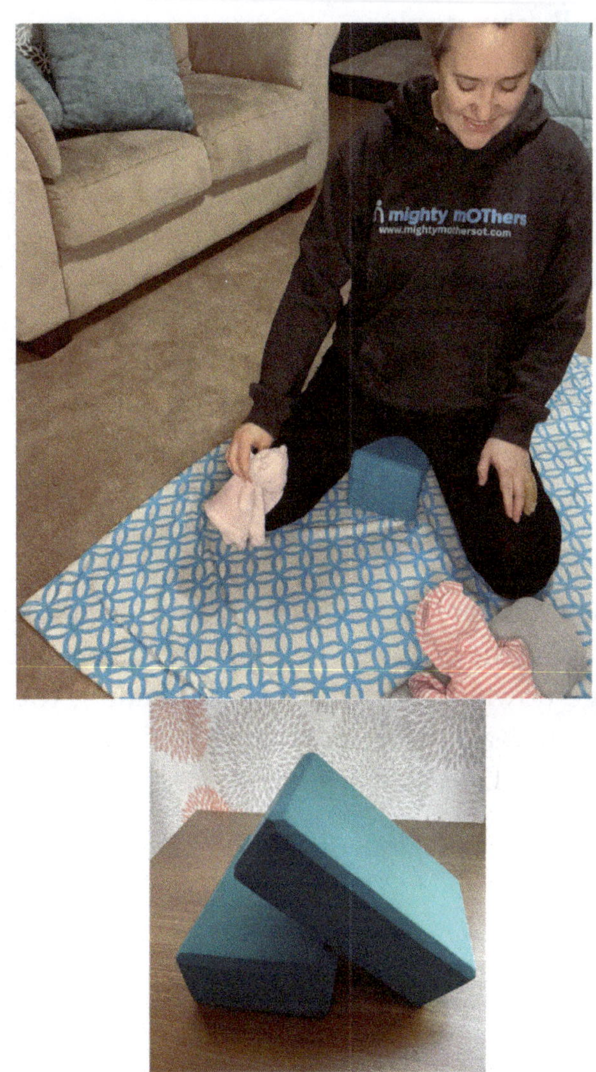

Small step stool:

That first postpartum poo can be a doozy, but this can help! Get your pooping anatomy set up for better success. By propping your feet up and getting your knees higher, the angles of your innards are much more conducive for flowing (and can better use gravity to move things along), which keeps the poo moving efficiently and with less strain. This will also help protect your pelvic floor. This goes for the first poo after baby comes, and onward from there. They do sell stools specifically for this purpose, but you can also consider using a stack of books or a toddler stool to get your feet and knees up in a pinch! To spread the legs for a more comfy position (keeping the belly area in mind as swelling takes time to go down and the scar may be tender), you could even use a combo of a stool and an overturned trashcan. Do what ya gotta do!

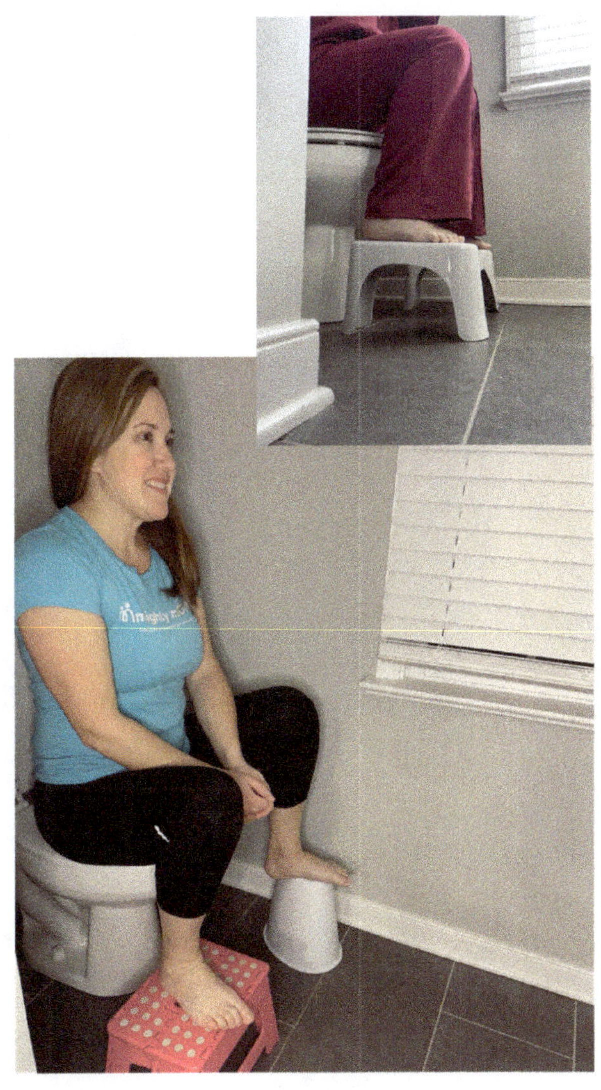

52

5
WHEN ALL ELSE FAILS: BREATHE

We already breathe a lot of times per hour, every single day, so what gives, you may ask?! There are actually a few simple, but important, strategies to use to get full, deep, cleansing breaths. This is super important anytime, but especially after giving birth, and especially after having a major surgery.

The baby grew, and your body grew and shifted to accommodate baby. Because you sort of ran out of room, you probably stopped taking in full, deep breaths and got used to using "accessory" muscles to help you breathe. Your posture likely also changed, which can greatly affect the amount of oxygen you are pulling in when you take a breath. And of course, once you have your surgery, you may be "guarding" yourself from taking deep breaths, worried about the (very real) pain from moving too much or too quickly.

One big reason for working on your breathing is to relearn how to breathe properly, now that things have mostly gone back to their place and your scar is beginning to heal. Using your big, appointed breathing muscles is better than relying on accessory muscles: all that strain in your neck and upper back from breathing funny will go away, AND you'll protect your pelvic floor.

Breathing deeply and well also does a lot for decreasing stress. The diaphragm, when moving fully and properly during breathing, actually stimulates the vagus nerve. The vagus nerve is a huge part of our parasympathetic nervous system, which is our "rest and digest" system. Therefore, as the diaphragm works better and more, the vagus nerve works better and more, and you end up with more relaxation and stress reduction. What new mama doesn't want a little boost with that?!

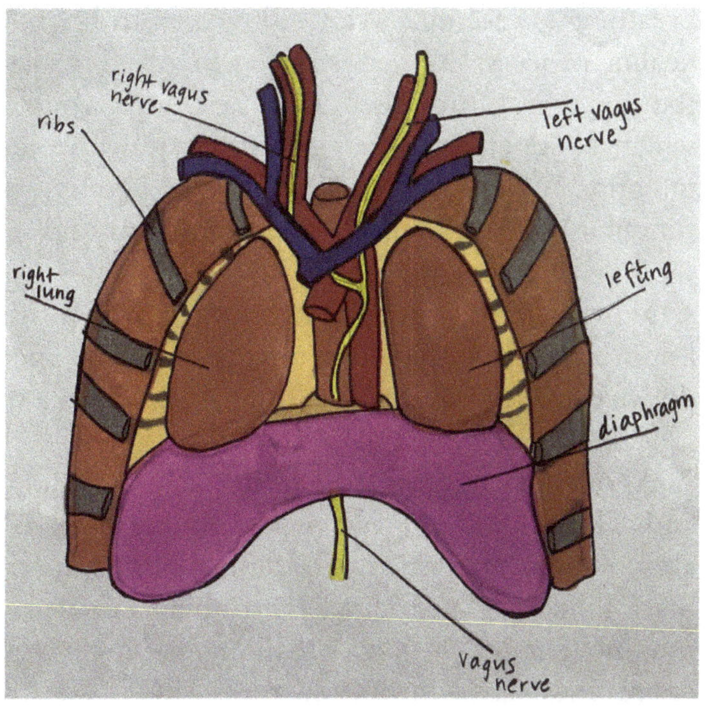

Pictured is a diagram that emphasizes the importance of 360 degree breathing – with an inhale, the lungs expand and the diaphragm moves downward, which hugs the vagus nerve. When the vagus nerve gets hugged, it fires off more signals for rest and relaxation.

As for C-section recovery, deep and full breathing is essential. We need oxygen to help the healing process. Oxygen is hugely involved in all of the biological processes that heal our wounds, which is super important for tissue function and integrity. When our tissues function better, we function better. Get that oxygen to that wound!

Now that I can step off my soap box about the importance of getting good oxygen efficiently, how do we do that?

A lot of us have heard about "belly breathing," and while that's not completely wrong, let's talk about an even better way to think about breathing. Start thinking "360-degree" breathing. You want the movement of your breathing to circle your entire chest area, in 360 degrees. This is because your lungs need lots of room to expand, and your ribs encircle your lungs. When you breathe in and out in a 360-degree pattern, you allow your ribcage to expand and contract in the front, sides, and back, and this gives your lungs plenty of room to do their thing.

Picture a small hula hoop or pool noodle circling your body, right at your ribcage. You want your ribs to expand fully to touch that noodle at all points in the front, back, and sides when you breathe in (and your lungs fill with air), and then shrink away from touching it at the front, back, and sides when you breathe out (and your lungs let the air out). Another helpful "cue" is to place both hands on your ribs, with your fingers pointing forward, and your thumbs pointing toward your back (fan your fingers out along your ribs, feeling where they are in the front, sides, and back). Tactile, or physical, cues like this help remind us what to do while we are learning something new.

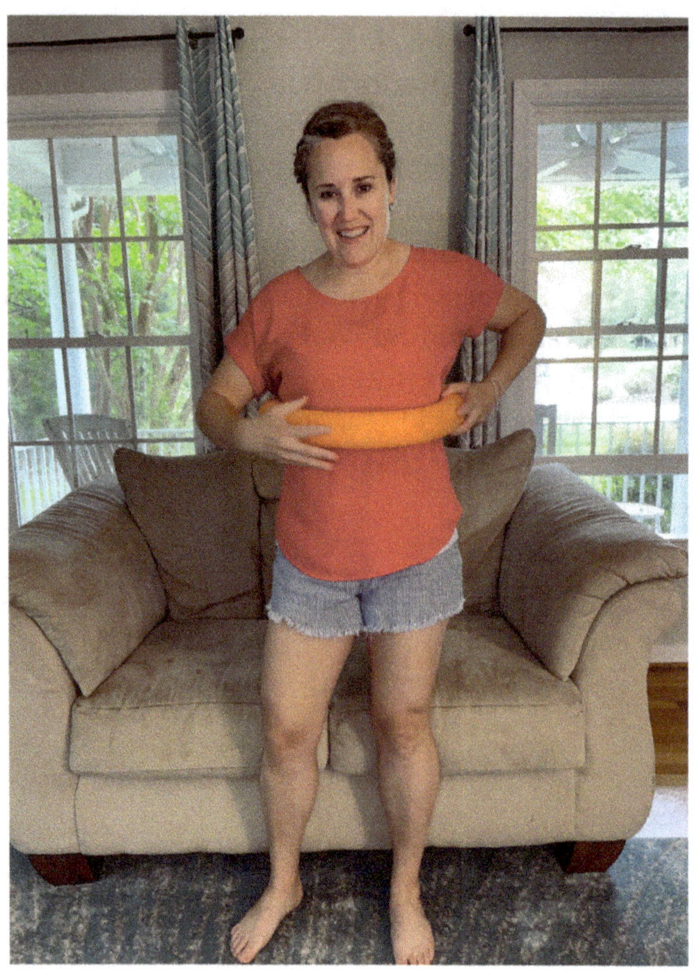

Breathing IN fully is generally more "active," or the "work" part of this process. But breathing OUT should be a completely relaxed movement, where the lungs are simply recoiling and pushing the air out without much, or any, effort.

If, at the beginning of healing, this causes any pain or discomfort, or if you are even simply worried that it might, grab a small pillow (or even a stuffed animal), and place it against your surgical area. Hug it to your scar while you practice breathing, to give you a little extra protection. Just make sure you are still focusing on the full expansion and relaxation part!

Though we do breathe all day, every day, try your best to incorporate 360-degree breathing into your daily life. Start with just 3 or 4 minutes a day and do it when you can focus ONLY on your breathing. Try it sitting or lying down first because your standing muscles will come more into play when you are standing or walking around, and it is harder to concentrate on breathing alone. Once you feel confident with this technique, throw it into your routine in more functional ways, such as when you go to stand up or sit down.

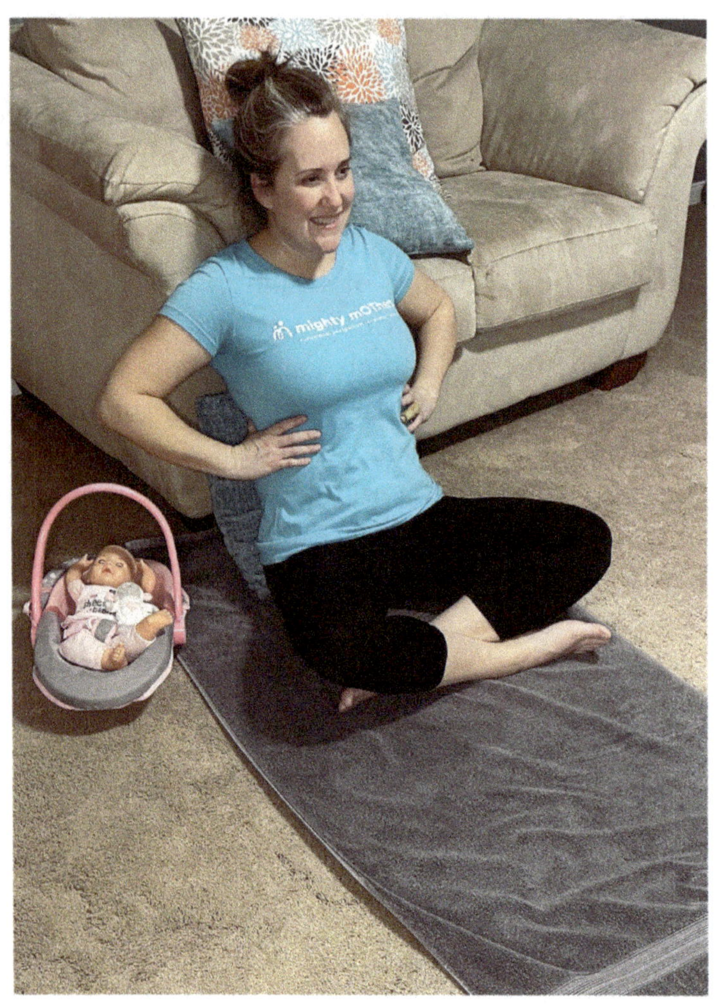

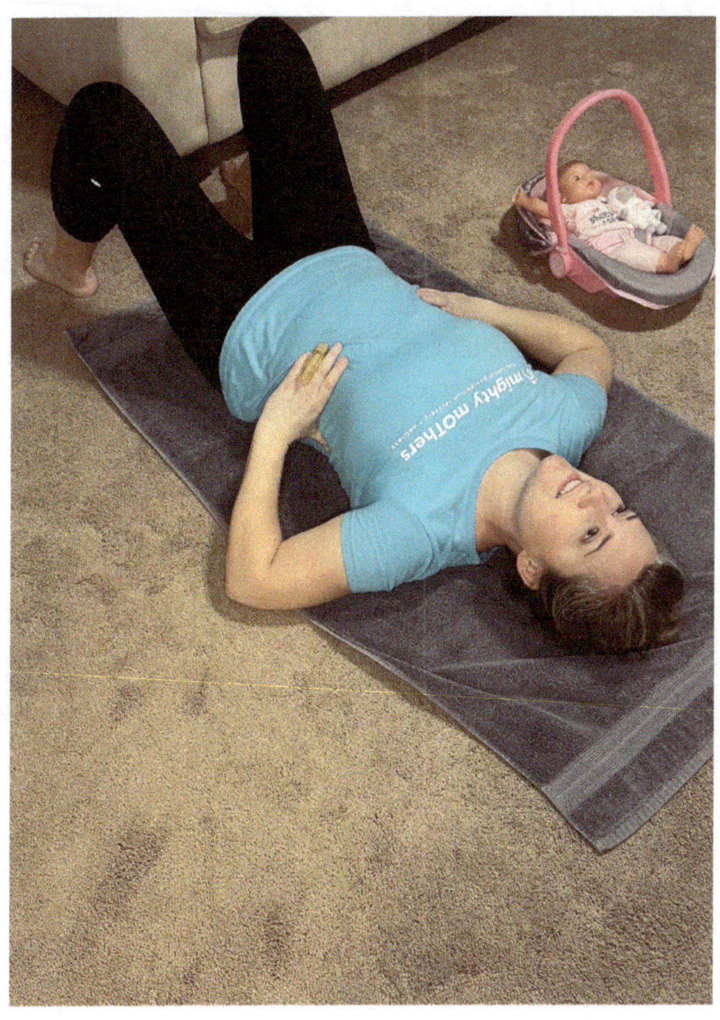
mighty mothers

Most important of all, work on exhaling as you exert yourself. Examples are: picking baby up while in the car seat carrier, placing baby into the sink or bathtub, and moving baby into the crib. Take a nice breath in first, then exhale slowly and with intention as you pick that carrier up. Take a breath in, then exhale as you lower baby into the crib. This will do wonders to protect your pelvic floor AND your healing C-section scar.

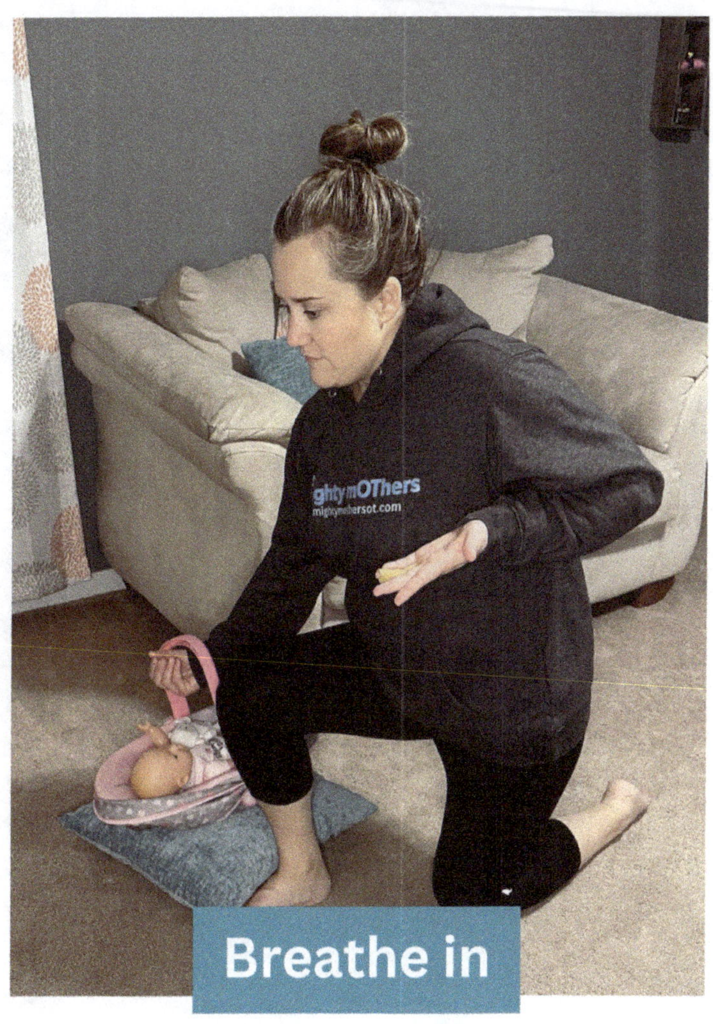
ghtymOThers
mightymothersot.com
Breathe in

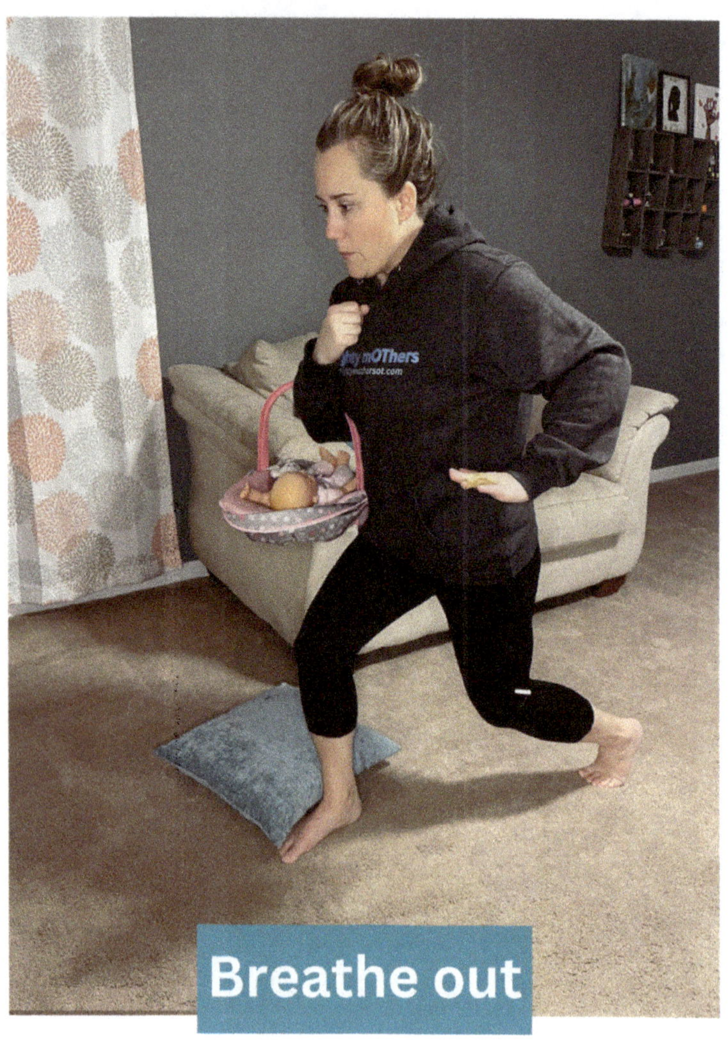
Breathe out

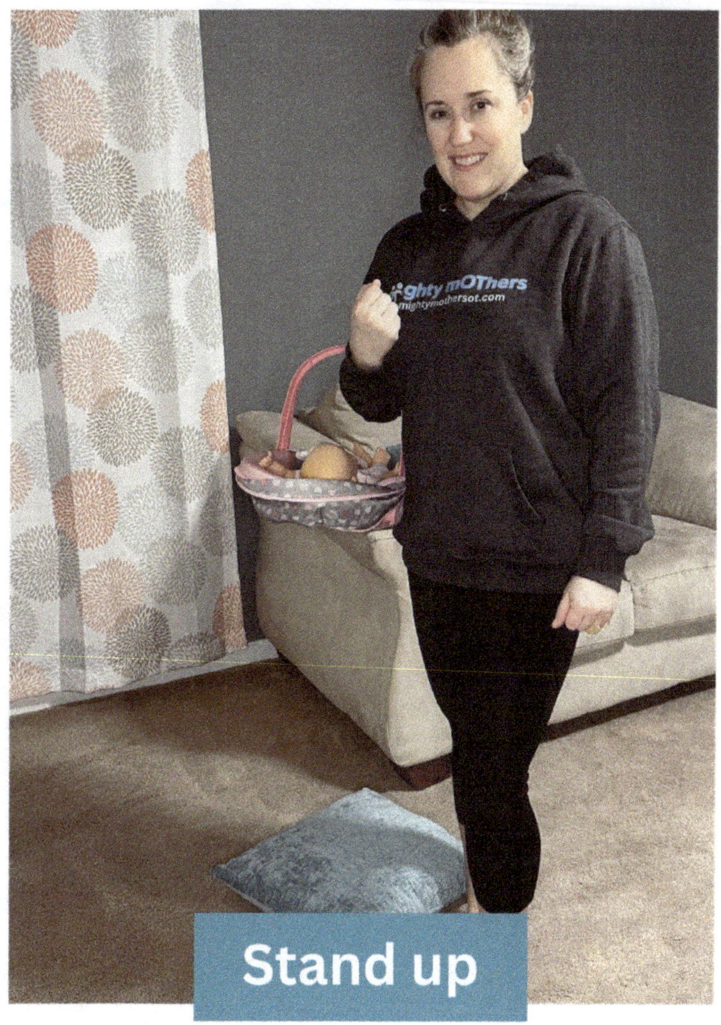
Stand up

6
SET GOALS AND EXPECTATIONS FOR YOU

When you start to consider your personal, unique recovery process, what do you see for yourself? Remember, just because the media portrays women "bouncing back" in certain, physically-focused ways, does NOT mean that has to be your one and/or only priority.

Think about what motivated you and inspired you before you had your baby, and before you went through this major operation. What is still important to you now? What is newly important to you now? Make a list! This may include physical aspects of your body, mental or emotional characteristics, activities you like to engage in, relationships you want to maintain, ways you like to participate in your house and community, etc.

Now, instead of setting goals to achieve an exact replica of the "Before C-Section You," is there a way to use Before C-Section You as a guide, but not a hard and fast guideline? Can you set goals that work toward a stronger, more rested, less mentally foggy you than the Immediately After Surgery You?

Your body and mind have just gone through a major change. A conversation I've had many times with my patients and clients is about this: your body and mind simply aren't the same as they once were, so it's unfair to compare them at this moment to how they were before your surgery and the birth of your baby. It's like comparing apples to oranges, as they say. Remember: different doesn't always, or only, mean bad!

Another thing to consider during the healing process is the type of body and mind you had before your birth and major surgery. Were you more sedentary, or fairly active? What was your pain tolerance like before this surgery? How did you process and cope with change and stress before the birth of your baby?

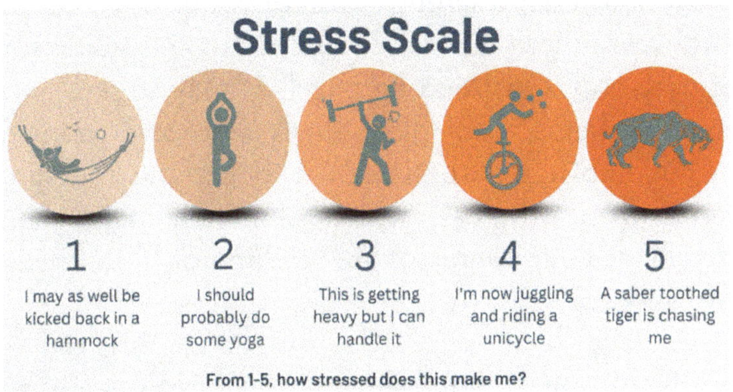

Knowing the answers to some of these questions can help you set realistic goals and expectations, and help you avoid reinventing the wheel with your healing and recovery.

When you are setting goals for yourself, go ahead and write them down (see the end of this guide for a very cool Goal Setting page!) It may sound silly, but it helps you plan them out and remain accountable. It also REALLY helps you measure your own progress, which ultimately helps you decide if your strategies are working or if you need to shift gears.

Think about how you can take baby steps to achieve the goals you have set for yourself. For example, instead of forcing yourself to immediately walk 3 miles a day, maybe a baby step goal could be something like "I will walk around my living room 20 times today." The next day could be 25! Before you know it, you will think that's super easy and you'll be ready to move along and challenge yourself some more. Also, think about (and write down!) what motivates you. Being as specific as you can helps your brain keep connecting with your goals to help you stay on track.

Consider how you will measure your own success. Can you count how many times you accomplished a particular task in a day? Or can you assess yourself on a 1-5 scale? (For example, "On a scale of 1-5, with 1 being not great and 5 being awesome, how well did I do attending to my own basic needs today?" or "On a scale of 1 to 5, how much did pain interfere with my life today?") Seeing a pattern of real "data" can help you see progress and help shift your mindset more positively about the efforts and progress you truly are making.

Progress Tracker	
Date	**Progress** 1-5 (5 is worst pain)
10/5	Scar pain - 5 (can't do anything today)
10/6	Scar pain - 3 (able to take short walk)
10/7	Scar pain - 4 (took a shower)
10/8	Scar pain - 3 (stood for doing dishes)

Remember, each individual has his/her own set of priorities, and reasons behind them. There should be no judgment for what you focus your energy on as you transition from pregnancy to new mama after a major surgery. Think about and write down what motivates you - after all, what motivates you ultimately helps you be more successful and focused!

Think about any possible barriers to your accomplishing the baby steps you will use to work toward your bigger goals for your C-section recovery. Are you overwhelmed, too tired, or don't know how to get things done with baby around? Then think of what you can do to get past those barriers. Can you delegate some things to someone else, do something while baby is doing tummy time, or write out a priority list to take away some overwhelm? Cross off each barrier as you barrel through it - it will feel so good!

Roadblocks: Write 'em down, cross them off!

~~My C-section scar hurts and moving around scares me~~

The baby cries a lot

I can't find the time to take care of myself

Try to keep in mind you did undergo a major surgery. Going slow and steady with your goals is a good thing - you want to prevent injury and pain, after all.

Rediscover your
mighty in
MOTHERHOOD

Goal-setting Planner

Big Picture Goal	**Baby Step Goal**	**Motivation**

Roadblocks: Write 'em down, cross them off!

Progress Tracker

Date	Progress

mighty mOThers

7

A FEW FINAL THOUGHTS

You've got this, mama! I hope you have found this information useful. Remember, protect yourself, and protect your peace and healing. You will feel better yourself, and you'll feel better and more confident as you step into your mama role. One day at a time, one small change at a time.

Check out the goal sheet below (there is an example, as well as a link to print your own), and print copies for your fridge so you can stick to your plan!

If you have specific concerns related to your healing and your body and mind, reach out to your healthcare provider (doctor or therapist). They have your healthcare records and know you and your background best, so they can make more specific suggestions related to your needs.

****

mighty mOThers, LLC was born when I realized how much I, myself, had struggled with C-section/postpartum recovery and saw firsthand how little support and information was out there for postpartum moms.

Today, mighty mOThers is proud to offer unique, important services to postpartum (and pregnant) mamas to get them the support and guidance they both need and deserve.

Check out more at www.mightymothersot.com, and consider subscribing to our newsletter for access to freebies, discount codes, and tons of useful information.

Important Links & Sources:

Goal-Setting Planner, Wellness Worksheet, and Mental Health Mantras:
www.mightymothersot.com/resources

Subscribe to our newsletter:
https://forms.wix.com/r/7062149711616016390

Article on Cesarean Deliveries:
Sung, Sharon, and Heba Mahdy, July 9, 2023. Cesarean Section.
https://www.ncbi.nlm.nih.gov/books/NBK546707/

Scan this code to check out the latest groups, classes, events, and more:

ABOUT THE AUTHOR

Natalie is a mom of two awesome kiddos, who both happened to be born via C-section. She's also an occupational therapist, with 15 years of experience and a passion for helping people find their function after surgery, illness, and trauma. Natalie began to focus on maternal health as an OT shortly after her own kids were born, related to her personal postpartum experiences, and her realization that there's a significant gap in care between pregnancy and postpartum when it comes to mamas.

Though Natalie's recoveries from each of her C-sections were slightly different (the first was an emergency and the second was planned), there was a common theme: she felt lost, alone, and uncertain about how to feel better mentally and physically - even though she was an OT! She wondered why there wasn't more support and information available.

As Natalie put together the information for this guide, she always had one main thought in mind: no mother should have to navigate this confusing and overwhelming recovery alone. Through sharing strategies and expertise as an OT and C-section mom, her dream is to inspire and uplift others so that every C-section mama feels confident and supported.

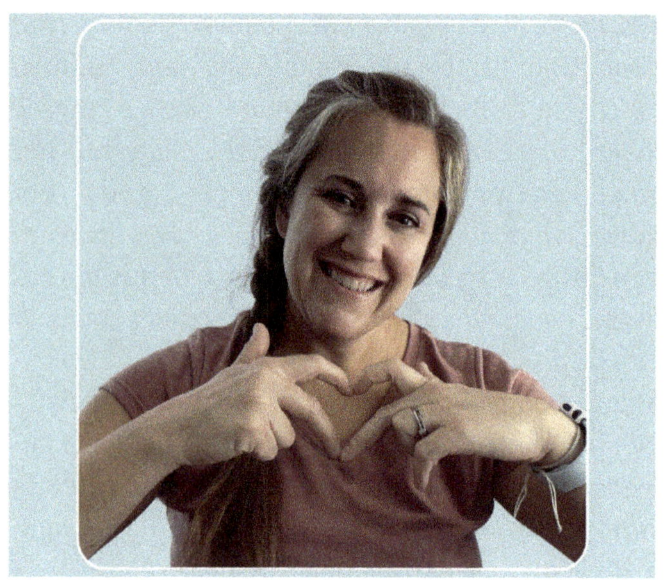